The Acid Alkaline Diet for Beginners

The Complete Guide Step By Step For Understand pH, Recipes And All Day Plan

By Laura Violet and Erika Sanders

Copyright © 2019

All right reserved. No portion of this book may be reproduced, stored in a retrieval system, or transmitted in any form or by any means – electronic, mechanical, recording or otherwise – except for brief quotation in printed reviews without the prior written permission of the publisher or the author.

Legal Notices

No part of this publication may be reproduced or transmitted in any form or by any means, mechanical or electronic, including photocopying or recording, or by any information storage and retrieval system, or transmitted by email without permission in writing from the publisher.

While all attempts have been made to verify the information provided in this publication, neither the author nor the publisher assumes any responsibility for errors, omissions, or contrary interpretations of the subject matter herein.

This publication is not intended for use as any source of advice such as legal, medical, or accounting. The publisher wants to stress that the information contained herein may be subject to varying international, federal, state, and/or local laws or regulations.

The purchaser or reader of this publication assumes responsibility for the use of these materials and information.

Adherence to all applicable laws and regulations, including international, federal, state and local governing professional licensing, business practices, advertising, and all other aspects of doing business in the US, Canada or any other jurisdiction is the sole responsibility of the purchaser or reader.

Table of Contents

INTRODUCTION 4

CHAPTER ONE 5

    WHAT IS ALKALINE DIET? 5

        Myths about Alkaline Diet 7

        Why Alkaline Diet? 19

        What to Do if it Doesn't seem to Work? 24

CHAPTER TWO 29

    ALKALINE FOODS THAT HELP YOU LOSE WEIGHT 29

CHAPTER THREE 52

    ARE YOUR FOODS ACIDIC? 52

        What are problems with an acid-forming diet? 53

CHAPTER FOUR 60

    HOW TO MAKE THE BODY MORE ALKALINE – AND LESS ACIDIC 60

        How does your Body become more Alkaline? (or more Acidic) 60

        Ways to Make Your Body More Alkaline 61

        What is the link between the alkaline diet and cancer? 78

CHAPTER FIVE 81

Alkaline Recipes that you Should Try Out 81

CHAPTER SIX 113

How to Start an Alkaline Diet plan 113

Sample day: Alkaline diet plan 116

CHAPTER SEVEN 122

Is my favorite sauce alkalizing? 122

CONCLUSION 128

Introduction

Over the years, we have had a lot of meal lifestyles crop up, from the Atkins diet to the Ketogenic diet, and out of all of them, only the Alkaline diet stands out. It has been so effective in improving bone health, teeth health, and even shedding weight to the extent that A-listers such as Hollywood Stars are lovers of it.

Why are they crazy about the Alkaline diet? Is it true that the Alkaline diet has been rumored to help treat cancer or even prevent it?

We will analyze everything that you need to know about the Alkaline diet; its benefits, meal plan and so on. Just read on.

Chapter One

What Is Alkaline Diet?

An alkaline diet may be defined as different things by different people, but the basis of the diet is that the acidic foods that one consumes, which wreak havoc in the body, should be tossed away for alkaline foods, as they improve your health.

You may be wondering how this works. It is quite simple. When the pH of the body is controlled to an extent, there is a great chance that your body will appreciate you for it by being healthy, losing weight, and preventing terminal ailments such as heart disease and cancer.

Controlling the pH level does a lot more, as it is excellent in skin care routines. Some beauty experts advise those that want glowing skin to alter their diet to include more Alkaline, and cut down on acidic foods.

The pH level has a ranking from one to fourteen. If you fall below seven, that means you consume a lot of acidic foods such as dairy, animal fats and vinegar.

If you fall above seven, that means you consume a lot of alkaline foods, which are mostly plant-based foods. Usually, when food is digested, what is left over is either alkaline and acidic, which is sometimes called ash. When you dive into the world of the alkaline diet, you may hear it being called the alkaline ash diet.

Having more acidic ash in the body than alkaline ash isn't great for it.

According to proponents of the alkaline diet, acidic ash can be dangerous to your health. T0 curtail this, you have to try out an affordable system to curb the level in the body.

Myths about Alkaline Diet

Can changing my diet affect my health?

This is the basic truth. Why do you think health experts advise that if you want to eat healthily, you should watch what you consume? It is common to see them advise one to avoid junk foods, animal-based foods, and have them focus on plant-based foods.

Have you noticed that vegans lead a healthier lifestyle than one that munches on any food that comes across their table? Leading a vegan lifestyle isn't easy, and a lot of people end up cheating because it is stringent. That's why the alkaline diet should be something that you should consider.

For someone that wants to shed weight, reducing the calories you consume is essential, and the alkaline diet is the way forward.

I have seen a lot of people mumble about taking a lot of miracle pills, but at the end of the day, nothing seems to be working. A lot of pills bought off the shelf barely work. Only a few are known to help, and even after that, your diet matters. You can't be taking miracle fat shedding pills, expecting them to work, and munching on foods that are high in calories and cholesterol.

What of those that go to the gym a lot, yet nothing seems to be working? It is common to see a lot of people sweating themselves regularly at the gym, but instead of shedding weight, they are gaining rapidly. It shouldn't make you feel like exercising doesn't work. It does, but is your diet cooperating with the exercise routine? You can't be exercising and taking diets that are not in line with your weight shedding principles. It is a complete waste of time.

An alkaline diet can help improve your bone and teeth health, shed weight, and even prevent cancer, as well as other terminal ailments.

Is the Alkaline Diet Healthy?

If you are asking this question, then the answer is a resounding 'yes.' The alkaline diet is one of the healthiest diets known to man. Why is this so?

For you to be on an alkaline diet, then you should have removed processed meats from the list of things that you consume. Do you know that a lot of processed meats lead to cancer? These same processed meats are listed amongst the foods that adherents of alkaline diet should avoid since they have high acidity.

What an alkaline does is to help balance the pH level, and it can be done when a person eats a lot of alkalizing foods like veggies and fruits. This also involves removing highly acidic foods like refined grains and processed meats.

If these aren't healthy, what else is then?

Will I lose weight?

Trying the alkaline diet can make you shed weight. This is guaranteed, as it is designed to restrict the number of calories that you consume. The foods that are high in calories are avoided and replaced with veggies and fruits. You may decide to consume a bit of both, but the veggies and fruits should top all.

When you consume those healthy foods, you will realize that weight loss becomes the goal. Before you know it, you will have the body of your dreams without even hitting the gym. Isn't that great?

Is it good for the teeth?

Do you know that alkaline diets are great for the teeth? How is this possible? Your mouth's pH level is heightened using the saliva, and it increases your oral health.

Do you know that acidic foods can destroy the teeth? The consumption of acidic foods mostly causes plaque.

Before you know it, you are battling with one oral issue or the other, and your smile's health is affected as a result. Acidic reflux caused by consumption of highly acidic foods is said to be the cause of the tooth enamel eroding. Consume alkaline foods, and you will be surprised by how your smile improves.

Can an Alkaline Diet Improve Bone Health?

This question bears a similar answer with the rest, 'yes.' Research has shown that eating foods that are high in acid can lead to the calcium in your bones being eroded. This is because calcium works to balance the pH of the body.

Basic chemistry class taught us that calcium is a base, and it can easily neutralize acid. The body has a state that it gets to which unleashes calcium to neutralize acid.

This means that if you eat a lot of foods that are high in acid, the calcium in your bones will be used to neutralize it.

Other factors work together to determine the level of calcium that is removed from the bones.

Proof shows that eating foods high in alkaline can reduce the amount of calcium that is removed from the bones to neutralize acidity. Foods like alcohol and coffee should take the back seat in your diet, according to the National Osteoporosis Foundation.

Can an Alkaline diet improve heart health?

When we talk about the heart, we can only say that we have to be careful with what we consume. The heart is a delicate part of the body, and comes with a lot of functions, meaning that if the heart is not working, the other parts of the body are doomed. Some foods are called heart-healthy foods, and acidic foods are far from being on the list.

If you want your heart to be healthy, you should consider eating a lot of plant-based foods.

Since the alkaline diet doesn't have the processed meat and animal protein factors, you won't have to worry about your body being laced with a lot of sodium. Sodium has been linked to an increase in blood pressure in the body.

Do you know that consuming foods that are high in alkaline helps to take off those waistline saboteurs like sweets and processed foods?

Those that are obese and have high blood pressure are at a higher risk of developing heart disease. An alkaline diet helps to reduce those risk factors, thereby improving your heart health.

Can an alkaline diet reduce cancer risk?

A lot of foods that are ranked as cancer-fighting are mostly alkaline diet foods. Yes, you read that right. If the foods that doctors advise those that want to prevent cancer from taking are alkaline foods, shouldn't that tell you that an alkaline diet is efficacious against cancer development?

For foods that are based on plants, they are excellent in reducing the risk of one developing cancer, and a lot of cancer survivors will advise that you try them. This is based on research by the American Cancer Research Institute.

The University of Alabama at Birmingham released its research on cancer and showed that consuming a plant-based diet was great in treating a variant of breast cancers that are said to be very dangerous.

Some drugs work much better in an alkaline environment than they do in an acidic environment.

Before you try out the alkaline diet, it is important that you consult your doctor if you are treating cancer.

Will an alkaline diet improve back pain?

A lot of people feel back pain regularly. It is common to see people take a lot of pills to treat back pain, and they realize that they are addicted to the pills, yet they are not working. Instead of pumping yourself with a pills that may turn out to be harmful, you should try out the alkaline diet. A lot of things cause back pain, but a major reason is an acid-rich diet.

Studies have shown that those with chronic back pain felt a lot better when they consumed an alkaline supplement that had magnesium — those who didn't, still had a backache. The alkaline supplement helped to neutralize the acid that was causing the backache, and before they knew it, their muscles were relaxed, and the pain had diminished greatly.

Losing Weight with an Alkaline Diet

When we talk of losing weight, we can say it is one of the most lucrative niches in the health industry. A lot of people spend money to shed weight, and that's why you see a lot of pills selling. If it is not people trying out slimming pills, it is slimming tea or a slimming belt. The options are numerous, and at the end of the day, one may realize that many of them do absolutely nothing.

If you have decided to lose weight, it is advisable to try out natural methods by eating healthy via an alkaline diet, exercising, and reducing the stress in your life.

When a lot of people try out the alkaline diet, they realize that weight loss is one effect they notice. There are others that nothing seems to work for the way they want it to. They may have lost weight with the Alkaline diet, but not the way they want. There are a few of these people, and I have noticed that their problem stems from other aspects of their lives. They would have reached their goals if they had slept better and reduced the stress they felt. The alkaline diet works like magic, but are you giving it the needed environment to work?

Losing weight also comes with another effect, becoming healthier, and this can be made possible with an alkalizing hydration regime, exercise, and diet. Before you know it, you are losing excess fat and leading a healthy life.

Too Heavy or Too Thin!

Over time, I have heard some people compliment the effect that an alkaline diet offers them. They shed weight quickly, unlike other methods that they have used. Some are great with their shape, while others overdo it, and become a lot thinner.

Did you know that the reason for trying an alkaline diet is to help lead a healthy life, and losing weight is an aspect of that? The aim of the alkaline diet is not to restrict yourself until you become thin, but to re-balance the pH and have your body re-energized.

Why an Alkaline Diet?

When the acidity level in the body increases, the body deals with it by increasing its weight. Did you know that as you merely exist, the body produces lots of acid? Consuming acidic foods worsens this.

At this point, you are overburdening your body, and it has to adapt. What does it do? It starts to gain weight.

As the acids get out of control, you start noticing that the body starts storing more fatty tissue. This is why you need alkaline foods. The fact that the body produces acid on its own means that it needs alkaline to neutralize it. When you consume alkaline foods, you are neutralizing the effects of acid.

Have you ever listened to those that have shed weight via an alkaline diet? What did you notice? There is a great chance that they all sounded dramatic because it is true. The alkaline diet worked magic, where other foods and weight loss methods couldn't. All of them have stories like eating a lot of green plant foods like wheatgrass, cucumbers, chard, watercress, kale, spinach, parsley, as well as those green leaves that are seen on the top of the beetroot.

The plant foods listed above have the following weight normalizing qualities like:

They have little sugar. Consuming foods high in sugar has been linked to obesity. Why do you think doctors advise people to avoid foods that are high in carbs? If you want to shed weight, you should consider minimizing your intake of sugar and increasing your intake of alkaline foods.

They have a lot of nutrients. These foods have lots of minerals and vitamins that greatly improve how the body functions. If you want an energized and healthy body, you should consider increasing your intake of alkaline foods.

When you eat them raw, you will notice that these foods come with a lot of negative charge, or electrons. This makes the energy in the body flow well.

Plant-based foods are reservoirs of large quantities of magnesium, which is great in improving the way the heart pumps, thereby removing the unwanted matter. Once you eat a lot of magnesium-containing foods, you will realize that you will lose a lot of waste that clogs up the body.

These foods have high chlorophyll, which is important in building healthy red blood cells. To researchers, chlorophyll is one thing that helps to shed weight.

They have a lot of fiber. One thing that a lot of people that have put on a lot of weight lack is a large amount of fiber. Fiber is important as it helps the body to lose a lot of weight, instead clogging up the body. Not every source of fiber should be opted for, as some sources like apples and bran are known to be acidic.

Combating Weight Loss

A lot of people that have added many pounds did so mainly because of poor diet, and it is common to see them shying away from exercising. There is nothing wrong with that.

To help lose weight, especially when you don't have the strength to exercise, you should consider consuming a lot of greens and plant-based foods that are alkaline. You should also eat healthy fats, as well as salt, as they are energizing, and before you can say, 'Jack Robinson,' you are already agile and want to move around.

No one will have to tell you at that moment to exercise because you will have a burst of energy.

You should also consider trying out public transportation, as it is great for not only you but the planet, too.

What to Do if it Doesn't seem to Work?

A large number of those that have tried the alkaline diet have noticed the effects it has on shedding weight. In a few cases, it may not be working the way you want because something else in your life is canceling its effect.

If your consumption of alkaline foods has increased, and you are exercising, yet you are not getting what you want, you should try the following:

Are You Sleeping Well?

This is one question that you should ask yourself. It is common to see a lot of people think that when you sleep well, you increase in weight. This is a pure fallacy. The opposite is the truth. When you don't sleep well, you tend to gain weight because your body is stressed. Sleeping well allows your body to digest the food it has consumed, and you don't have to store up a lot of fat.

Are You Eating Late?

This is one question that you should answer. Do you belong to that school of thought that thinks eating late at night doesn't affect your metabolism? If you are, desist from it. You need to eat early enough to allow the body to digest the food on time, prevent you from being bloated. Eat your dinner before seven in the evening, no matter how busy you may be.

Are You Stressing Yourself?

Are you stressed? When the body is stressed, it increases the production of cortisol, a hormone that leads to the fattening of the body. A lot of people think that when they are stressed, they reduce in weight. The opposite is usually the truth. When you stress yourself, you will gain a lot of weight, and before you know it, you may be obese. When a person is fat, he or she tends to eat a lot. When you are stressed, what do you do? There is a great chance that it would be stuffing yourselves with sugar to feel good again. Try and remove the things that stress you from your life. If you can't remove them from your life, you should consider trying to de-stress yourself by using robust methods like yoga, massage and so on.

Are You Skipping Breakfast?

This is one wrong philosophy that a lot of people share. You see them skipping breakfast, thinking that it would help them shed weight, but usually, the opposite is the case. Instead of losing weight, they gain more. Did you know that when you skip breakfast, your body tends to overcompensate with what you eat for lunch? You will see yourself eating a lot during lunch and dinner. What then is the need?

How Are You Emotionally?

You may ask how this affects your weight. When you are feeling down, and you have no means of bringing yourself up, you may decide to rely on eating your way out of those unwanted feelings.

Do you feel that there is no purpose on earth for you? Or is something else pulling you down? You have to work on it if you want your weight loss to work.

Are You On Medication?

Not every medication you take is great with weight loss. Do you know that the drugs can be counteracting your weight loss? If you didn't know, now you do. When you take medications like oral contraceptives, there is a chance that losing weight may not be easy for you. The same can be said if you have a hormone-releasing device inside of you.

The drugs that you are taking are most likely acidic, hence why they can lead to weight increase. You should consider talking to your doctor to see if the dosage can be reduced.

Chapter Two

Alkaline Foods that Help You Lose Weight

For someone that wants to shed weight, and is considering trying out the alkaline diet, you should consider including these foods into your regular meals.

Before we continue, we can pretty much state that a lot of fruits and veggies are alkaline, even grapefruit and lemons.

You can also try organic eggs, organic meats, seeds, and so on, as they can help in shedding weight.

If you try these, you will notice weight loss. While on your journey to shedding weight via alkaline foods, you should consider reducing the number of refined foods that you consume. Toss fast foods, beverages or snacks to the garbage can. High alkaline foods are not only good but also great for the taste buds.

Some things that you should consider adding in your meal plan while trying out the alkaline diet are:

Herbs:

Herbs are great alkaline ingredients that can be used to flavor the foods. They are also great in shedding weight.

Beverages:

While losing weight using the alkaline diet, you need a lot of liquid, and that's where beverages come into play. This doesn't mean that you should consume sugary ones.

Other snacks:

Who said you couldn't munch on snacks because you are trying an alkaline diet? The only thing that you should avoid are snacks that are high in carbs. There are snacks available that are tasty to the taste buds and are low in carbs.

Carb and sugary substitutions:

We all love sweet things and denying ourselves of them can be difficult. You can consider taking sugary substitutions that do not have carbs and sugar. You will satisfy your taste buds and shed weight.

This isn't the entire list of things that you should take on the alkaline diet; we have decided to mention only a few. There are a lot more that can be used to shed weight.

    i.   Alkaline Water

A lot of fruit juices and sodas out there have a lot of sugar. They should be avoided because they go against the tenets of the alkaline diet. It is important that you keep your body hydrated with water, and not soda or fruit juices. You can take fruit juices, only when they don't contain sugar, and they aren't made from overly acidic fruits.

You should also consider hydrating yourself with alkaline water. You are guaranteed to shed weight and still benefit from the pros of alkalizing. With the alkaline water, you are sure to lead a healthy life and still lose weight.

ii. Almonds and Almond Milk

When it comes to nuts, almonds are some of the healthiest known to humanity. If you want to lead a healthy lifestyle, especially one with an alkaline diet, you should try almonds. Almonds are awesome because they help to reduce the level of cholesterol in your body.

They can act as a great snack, instead of snacks that are high in calories. You should toss out those chips that are high in calories, and opt for almonds. If you want milk, you should consider almond milk, as it is an awesome substitute for dairy milk. It tastes almost like dairy milk, and you can use it, to a large extent, for what dairy milk is used for.

iii. Artichokes

Have you eaten artichokes? If you have, you are in luck as you can introduce Folates and Vitamins K and C into the body. They come with a lot of antioxidants as well. They are also great for fighting off free radicals.

You can use them in a lot of dishes like salad to get that additional flavor. They also make a great dip. Research has shown that artichokes function as a liver purifier, and are great for digesting foods.

iv. Avocados

Avocados! These are one of the best things that Mother Nature gave to humanity. If you want to alkalize the pH of your body, you should consider incorporating avocados into your meal. A lot of researchers have christened, 'avocado,' as the superfood anyone who wants a healthy life should consume regularly.

For those that eat a lot, have problems filling up, and always feel hungry, avocados can help. How is this possible? Due to containing oleic acid, avocados will quench your hunger quickly.

This means that you won't be hungry easily, and won't eat a lot more than is needed. That's not all, remember we said that avocado is a superfood.

Avocados possess healthy fats or LDL fats that help to reduce the level of cholesterol in your body. If you want your metabolism rate to be heightened, you should consider taking a lot of avocados. When your metabolism rate increases, you tend to shed weight quickly.

Avocados come with anti-cancer benefits. Research has been linked with avocados and their ability to prevent cancer to a large extent. Avocados are also anti-inflammatory, meaning that eating a lot of avocados helps to reduce your risk of getting inflammations.

That's not all, as you can see avocados in a lot of delicious recipes. Who said you have to give up healthy and delicious foods? You can't use salad dressings while on an alkaline diet. Try to substitute them for avocado oil, as it does the trick, and it is healthier. There are still some salad dressings that are great for an alkaline diet, but not all of them.

v.   Beets

It is common to see a lot of people ignoring beets in their diet. If you are one of them, you need to rectify the mistake by adding more beets to your diet.

They are great at increasing the pH level in your body, thereby reducing the acidic nature of your body.

That's not all, as beets come with betalains. Betalains have been linked with fighting cancer and have been called cancer-fighting phytonutrients. The beets can be steamed if you want, or you can add them to that smoothie you are making.

You should consider opting for fermented beets, as their natural sugar is consumed while fermentation occurs. The bacteria eat it up, offering you beets devoid of sugar.

Beets are great sources of beneficial enzymes, as well as healthy probiotics.

You can use the fermented beet powder in smoothies. It doesn't have the taste of the fermented beets, meaning that you can drink healthy smoothies.

vi. Bell Peppers

Many great dishes contain bell peppers. Bell peppers are loved by many people and come in many different hues. They can be eaten in a lot of foods, and your body thanks you for giving it foods that have bell peppers. Their health benefits are out of this world, as they have hydroxycinnamic acids, flavonoids, and carotenoids.

They act as anti-inflammatories and can help to minimize joint inflammation. For those that have diabetes, consuming them helps a lot. What of those that want their cardiovascular system improved? Bell peppers help, and they are high in alkaline.

Bell peppers are also called superfoods, as they have a lot of Vitamin C. They have more vitamin C than oranges. The significant aspect is that they possess a lot of vitamin C, without as much sugar as in oranges.

You can't get the necessary vitamin C for the body to function only through bell peppers, and that's why we advise that you try out vitamin C supplements.

vii. Bok Choy

For those that are lovers of Asian foods, there is a great chance that you know Bok Choy, and you love it. This food has a lot of nutrients, especially Vitamins K, C, and A. That's not all, as Bok Choy is an excellent source of folate and fiber.

Did you know that it also contains phenolic compounds? Phenolic compounds are known to help fight off damage caused by free radicals. Bok Choy also comes with omega-3 fatty acids.

A lot of people use Bok Choy in stir fry, but it is used for much more. You can eat it raw and even add it to soups and stews.

viii. Broccoli

There are hardly any people that haven't eaten broccoli. We ate it from childhood, and some of us were forced to eat it. If you want to heal well, you need to eat a lot of broccoli. Broccoli has a lot of uses and can be used in multiple ways.

Broccoli can also be considered a superfood. If you want the rate of your metabolism to increase, you need it. When your metabolism increases, you lose weight quickly. It is awesome for one's immune system, as well as the digestive system.

Have you stared at broccoli sprouts and wondered why they are green? Don't be surprised, as they are known to have a lot of nutrients. Consuming the mature ones will give you a large amount of sulfuraphane.

You can decide to grow broccoli sprouts in your backyard. It is quite easy to do, and you can save money. It comes fresh and even organic. Isn't that great?

ix. Cantaloupe

For those that are used to cereals, you can toss them in the trash can. For those who don't think their breakfast is complete without the morning toast that has a lot of carbs, you are in luck. Cantaloupes can help. They are very nutritious and come with great taste. If you want to have the right amount of vitamins B6 and C, you should try cantaloupes. They also possess a high amount of potassium.

x. Cayenne Pepper

For those that are wondering why we added cayenne pepper to the list, let's take it slowly. Did you know that cayenne pepper is great for increasing your metabolic rate? We all know that as the metabolism increases, your body sheds weight. If weight loss is your plan, you should think of adding cayenne pepper to your diet.

Cayenne pepper is great for adding flavor to your meals. Cayenne pepper makes your food delicious; can't we say that it is a clear example of killing two birds with one stone? It is awesome in helping to fight off free radicals and helps to provide vitamins. You can add it to your soups, stews, salads, as well as eggs.

xi. Celery

When we talk of alkaline foods, the list can't be complete if we don't add celery. It is not only alkaline, but it is also a great source of water to keep you hydrated while you shed weight, as well as electrolytes. If you want a food that is high in Vitamins K and C, you should try out celery.

For those that want to shed weight, you don't have to stress yourself, as it possesses phthalides. Phthalides are great in reducing the amount of cholesterol in the body.

Research has shown that celery helps in reducing one's blood pressure. This means that if you are suffering from high blood pressure, you should try celery.

Try out celery in any meal at all, and you will benefit from the added alkaline. You can decide to eat it alone or can put it in juice, soups, as well as stews.

xii. Coconut Oil

Once you start to adhere to the alkaline diet, you should try to cut down on your usage of vegetable oils. You consider trying out coconut oil, as it is a great alternative if you want to reduce your intake of fats.

When we talk of natural alkaline oil, we have no other choice but to talk about coconut oil. It is known to be highly saturated and is great for cooking.

If you are thinking of trying coconut oil, you should opt for a virgin and organic one.

xiii. Cucumber

When you shed weight, you tend to lose a lot of electrolytes and water. What this means is that you need a source of hydration. What you need is cucumbers, as they are great sources of hydration. Not only do they offer the needed hydration, but they are also great for shedding weight.

A lot of people use cucumbers solely in salads, but it has a lot more usefulness than that. It can be used in stews and eaten alone. Cucumbers have a high content of antioxidants.

This is one food that has so many antioxidants that we have no choice but to call it the alkaline powerhouse. It also has nutrients like selenium, copper, phosphorus, magnesium, zinc, calcium, potassium, and vitamin C.

Studies have shown that cucumbers possess lignans. Lignans prevent the risk of one developing cancer.

    xiv.   Garlic

When it comes to losing weight, garlic helps quite a lot as well.

Garlic comes with a lot of benefits, and if we start listing them, it'll be hard to stop. It needs an eBook of its own to talk about how marvelous it is; no wonder the Asians are fascinated with it.

If you want to have your blood pressured reduced, you should consider taking more garlic. Garlic is said to help reduce the cholesterol level in one's body. If you want to prevent a lot of ailments like cancer, heart disease, flu, as well as bacterial infections, you should consider trying garlic.

Garlic can be added to a lot of foods because of the incredible flavor that it brings. Who doesn't like its aroma?

    xv.   Herbal Tea

Well, I had to add another beverage to the list, since we are taking away the usual beverages that a lot of people drink like black tea and coffee. Instead of taking coffee at the beginning of the day, you can consider using green tea or herbal tea as an alternative.

They have a high amount of alkaline and do not possess caffeine. One may scream in terror, but did you know that lacing your body with caffeine does more harm than good, as it increases your risk of getting high blood pressure.

Since herbal tea doesn't have caffeine, you won't be scared of your blood pressure increasing from consuming a lot of it. Instead, you tend to benefit from its weight shedding capabilities. Isn't that awesome?

They also come with a lot of health benefits. They're low in calories, anyone who wants to lead a healthy life should try them out. They are an awesome alternative to those juices that are sugary.

xvi. Kale.

Kale! What can we say about this awesome food? When you research the benefits of kale, you will be surprised. Kale is said to be a food that has a high content of alkaline. When it comes to the nutrients that kale has, you may be surprised. One of the nutrients that Kale has that we all need is potassium. Taking a serving of kale can give you the necessary potassium that you need in a day. Kale is said to help fight off cancer, and if you want your cholesterol level to lower, you should try it. Once you start using recipes with kale in them you'll realize how tasty it can be.

xvii. Lemons

When we say that lemons are alkaline, we get stares. "How can you say that lemons are alkaline?" they say. We aren't surprised that a lot of people feel that lemons are acidic because of how sour they are. When you consume lemons, and they are digested, they tend to be alkaline.

They possess a lot of vitamin C like oranges, but do not have as much sugar. You should consider adding lemon juice to your alkaline water, and it will feel like heaven on earth. It is great in reducing the level of cholesterol in your body as well.

xviii. Radishes

Radishes come in numerous forms, and all of them are known to be alkaline. They are known to have a lot of nutrients and contain a large amount of Vitamin C. The calcium in radishes is known to help prevent osteoporosis by reinforcing the bones. Like mentioned earlier, acidic food is known to force out calcium in the bone to neutralize it, but when you eat foods like radishes, you don't have to worry as much.

Radishes are low in calories, meaning that they are great alternatives for snacks that are high in calories, and they are great for shedding weight.

xix. Raisins

When it comes to dry fruits like raisins and apricots, they are very alkaline. Raisins are awesome sources of fiber, and we all know how important fiber is to the body.

That's not all, as raisins have a high amount of antioxidants. Antioxidants are needed to tackle free radicals. Raisins are great sources of other awesome nutrients like Vitamins B6 and B1.

For those that like to snack while watching a movie, you should consider snacking on raisins. You will fall head over heels in love with them.

xx. Spinach

For those that watched Popeye The Sailor Man, there is a good chance that you noticed the effects of spinach on that character.

When you are ranking alkaline superfoods, spinach is listed after kale as one of the best. It possesses a lot of nutrients that one needs like vitamin A, potassium, fiber, folate, iron, manganese, and magnesium.

It can be used in a lot of meals like eggs, salads, wraps, side dishes, pizza toppings, and even stir fry.

Chapter Three

Are Your Foods Acidic?

When we talk about eating alkaline, it means that you have decided to take your body from the slightly acidic stage to slightly alkaline. This means from 6.5 to 7.5.

A lot of foods that we consume tend to change the level of our pH. A lot of them when they have been digested, tend to leave a lot of harmful acidic by-products. As for those that are alkaline, they tend to leave behind alkaline by-products. Foods that can be called acidic are foods that have a high content of protein such as a lot of legumes like peas and beans, excluding lentils. Eggs, fish, and meat are also acid forming foods.

Foods like alcohol, coffee, and sugar are also acid-forming.

A lot of fruits and vegetables are alkaline foods. A lot of spices, seeds and nuts are also high alkaline.

Can we say that our ancestors did it right in the stone age, as they ate a lot of whole foods? They ate fish and game meat, but complemented them with a lot of roots, fruits, veggies, nuts, and seeds, giving them the right amount of pH — this is what they did for a long time before civilization started.

What are problems with an acid-forming diet?

If we could go back to the acid-alkaline balanced diet that those in the past ate, we would be better for it. Now, we only want to eat processed foods, grains, sugar, and a lot of other acid-forming foods. We eat less seeds, nuts, fruits and veggies that are alkaline forming. The way a lot of humans eat now has led them to suffer from 'chronic low-grade metabolic acidosis.'

The body may be designed to handle a bit of acid once in a while, but when it is continuous without the needed alkaline foods to neutralize it, we suffer for it. We end up depleting a large part of our alkaline reserves in the body and even eat down into the calcium in the bones.

If steps are not taken to have the acids neutralized, then the body suffers. You will have to deal with some health problems like osteoporosis. Many health issues can be tackled only if we ate more alkaline foods. Have you noticed that those who lived in the Stone Age that were able to survive war, drought and other environmental conditions did so because of their diet? Many of them lived for so long, without modern medicine.

Do you have signs of an "acidic" diet?

Some people have asked me how they can tell if they are currently eating a lot of acidic diets.

It is quite easy to tell if you are currently eating a lot of acidic foods if you look at the content of the food. We have already discussed some alkaline foods, as well as their acidic counterparts. The content of your food can help you see if it is acidic or alkaline. Apart from the content of the food, if you notice the following symptoms, it means that you are eating foods that have high acidic content:

- Weight gain

Are you one that has noticed weight gain, and nothing you do to shed the weight is working? There is a good chance that a large part of the food you consume is acidic. It is common to see people taking a lot of pills, using slimming belts and even exercising, but instead of shedding weight, they are gaining it. This is where alkaline foods can help. Once you cut down on the acidic foods and eat more alkaline foods, you will notice a loss of weight.

- Nonspecific aches and pains, especially in the bones and joints

This is one common symptom in those that consume a lot of foods that are high in acid. Normally, the body produces acid, and when you eat foods that are high in acidic content, it overburdens the body with a high content of acid that it has to neutralize. What does it do? To cope, it starts looking for alkaline to neutralize it. Calcium, in the bones, is a base that can easily neutralize the acid.

Before you can say, 'Jack Robinson,' your bone starts to suffer for it. This is why it is common to see those who eat a lot of acidic foods suffer from joint pains.

- Acid reflux or heartburn:

One problem a lot of people face is heartburn. It is common to see them squeezing their faces in pain because of it. This occurs because of acid reflux when you consume foods that are high in acidic content. Research has shown that foods that have high acidic content are known to lead to heartburn faster than foods that are high in alkaline. When the pH level of the body is acidic, the body suffers for it.

- Poor digestion, irritable bowels, intestinal cramping

Do you feel constipated? This can be caused by highly acidic foods because they aren't easy to digest, and many of them do not have fiber. Do you know that eating foods that are high in fiber can aid digestion? If you are someone that suffers a lot from poor digestion and intestinal cramping, then you should consider eating alkaline foods because they are high in fiber.

- Fatigue, feeling of being "run down."

A lot of acidic foods aren't as light as alkaline foods, and can't easily be digested. This is why you see a lot of people feeling tired easily. If you want to feel a burst of energy, you should consider eating foods that are high in alkaline content.

Other issues that can be faced when one eats foods that are high in acidic content are:

- Muscle weakness/loss of muscle
- Urinary tract problems
- Receding Gums
- Kidney stones
- Skin Problems

Chapter Four

How to Make the Body More Alkaline – and Less Acidic

By now, you must be wondering how you can turn your body into an alkaline one and reduce your level of acidity. We will analyze the various methods you can use, and you will increase the alkaline in your body in no time.

How does your Body become more Alkaline? (or more Acidic)

You may be wondering what ways your body becomes higher in alkaline or acid. There may be a lot of factors that determine the pH level of your body, but two main factors that lead to the body becoming alkaline or acidic are:

a. Foods That You Munch On

The foods that you eat regularly can determine the pH level in your body. If you consume foods like meats, soda, coffee, sugar, flour and chocolate a lot, your body tends to become acidic.

b. Your Stress Level

The way we stress our bodies can determine if they become acidic or not.

Ways to Make Your Body More Alkaline

We have discussed the issues that one can face from his or her body being acidic, meaning that you should consider working on getting an alkaline body. It may not seem easy, but the incredible benefits that you gain can help. Below are some strategies that can be used in turning your body into an alkaline one.

1. What is your pH level? Check it regularly.

This is something that you should regularly check because the pH level of your body can determine your state. You can check it yourself at home, without even taking a walk out of your room. There are pH strips that can be bought on Amazon, and they do not cost a lot. These strips can give you the needed readings, similar to if you had done the pH test in the hospital. You will easily tell what the alkaline and acidic levels of your body are.

From the results, you know what to do to ensure that your pH levels are balanced. When they are balanced, your body tends to have the important nutrients.

With these pH strips, you can easily check the levels of your pH at home. You should consider getting them. This test can be run via your urine or saliva. After fifteen seconds, you will see the test results. With the easy-to-read chart, you can tell what range you fall into.

2. Begin the day downing a large glass of water and a dash of lemon.

A lot of people tend to think lemons are acidic because of their sour taste, but the opposite is the case. Lemons are alkaline when they are digested. They are great in improving the rate of metabolism in your body. What you should do immediately when you wake up is to take clean water and add a dash of lemon. This gives you an effective energy boost that can do the trick.

When you take water and lemon, your body is given the needed energy via oxygenation and hydration. Want mental clarity and burst of energy? You should consider taking this daily when you wake up.

When you add a dash of lemon to water, the body becomes oxygenated, and the enzymes function well. Lemon helps to improve the function of the natural enzymes in the liver. If you want your liver to get rid of toxins effectively, like uric acid, then consider taking this combination.

3. Consume a lot of dark and green vegetables.

Remember those dark and green veggies that you may once have avoided? You should consider taking a lot more of them if you want to lead a healthy life, one where your body alkaline level is high.

Whenever I speak about healthy foods, my mind wanders to the hue green. The greener the food, the healthier one can say it is. Green is said to be the hue of life, and that isn't wrong. It is linked with nature.

When a people are deciding what to eat, the thought of eating green foods becomes scary. There are creative ways that green veggies can be incorporated into your diet without them coming across as being tasteless. We will discuss some creative recipes below.

The things that our taste buds are used to are mostly processed foods that are filled with lots of sugars and artificial flavors.

A lot of food producers have made us used to such flavors that a day without them makes us feel like we are about to give up the ghost.

If you are wondering how you can get your body to get adapted to green veggies, you should consider experimenting with them while you cook.

You can't tell which foods you will fancy until you eat them. You may think that you may hate the foods, but the opposite may be the case.

Instead of reaching up for potato chips or a bowl of ice cream, when you want to take care of your need for sweet things, you should consider taking cut up veggies. With time, you will love them.

4. Incorporating Exercise Routines

On your journey to shedding weight or staying healthy, you should consider exercising. Exercising can help make your body more alkaline, as you sweat out toxins. Combining exercise routines with alkaline foods can help get you in shape.

You don't have to be a gym rat before you exercise. You can take walks to the office instead of driving there. You can also cycle there. Try to swim regularly. If you are a great dancer, think of taking regular dance classes. What about yoga classes? They will leave you satisfied. You can also garden or take a walk with your loved ones or even pets. Once you exercise more, you will realize that the state of your health will improve. Your body needs exercise, give it to it.

When you exercise, you get the alkaline and acid balance that your body needs. As you grow your muscles, the high acidic content of the body reduces.

5. Reduce your alcohol intake.

When you consume alcohol a lot, your body's pH level changes, and becomes acidic. What this means is that your kidneys won't be able to function well because substances like phosphates can't be maintained in the bloodstream.

When the phosphates in your blood are imbalanced, it can lead to your body suffering from a slow metabolism.

As you drink alcohol, let's say a beer, you are taking a large amount of liquid and reducing the kidneys ability to remove it.

Before you know it, the levels of phosphates in your blood are altered.

A small bottle of alcohol can alter the functioning of a normal kidney. Alcohol also affects the liver, meaning that if your liver is damaged, the kidneys can suffer for it.

6. Drink a glass of water laced with natural baking soda

You are probably wondering if we are kidding you. The answer is 'no.' All you need to do when you wake up in the morning is to drink a glass of water that has a teaspoon of natural baking soda in it. It is a natural detoxifier.

When you drink it, brace yourself. It is not tasty, but your body will be alkalized quickly. This is an easy means of getting it done, and the effects are instantaneous.

There are a lot of benefits that it brings, but the major one is to have the pH levels of the body balanced. It goes a long way to improve your general wellbeing, while your energy is increased.

7. Reduce your intake of acidic foods.

One thing you should consider doing is restricting the intake of acidic foods that you consume. It can help in improving the levels of pH while improving the bone density. It also prevents the growth of kidney stones, as well as ridding oneself of the signs that come with acid reflux.

Those foods that are known to be an acidic need to be eaten moderately to prevent your acid level from increasing. The foods that fall under this category are pasta, walnuts, peanuts, eggs, processed cereals, bread, cake, cold cuts, oats, and rice.

As for beverages, try to avoid drinking a lot of milk, alcohol, drinks with a lot of sweeteners, as well as caffeinated drinks.

8. Consume a lot of alkaline water

There is a good chance that you have heard a lot of claims about what alkaline water offers. Alkaline water helps to do a lot of things, such as slowing the aging process. It can help in reducing the development of chronic ailments. That's not all, as it can control the level of pH in the body. Is it worth the hype? Let's see.

The alkaline water aids in neutralizing the acidic content in the body. When you take natural drinking water, you are consuming a liquid with a neutral pH of 7. As for the alkaline water, it comes with an alkaline pH of close to 8 or 9. You can search for alkaline water close to you.

9. Take a lot of multivitamins to supplement your diet.

Your body can easily be alkalized when you add vitamins to your diet. Vitamins C and A can help improve your immune system. That's not all, as it can strengthen the body's cells. Before you know it, your body will be alkalized.

Vitamin D is great in getting the body to an alkaline state and maintaining it. It is great in heightening calcium absorption, as well as improving the healthy mineral levels of the body.

A lot of these vitamins may not easily be consumed in the right quantity in our diets, but you should consider taking multivitamins. Before you know it, your pH level will be maintained.

10. Go for a brisk walk.

This is one routine that should be included in your life. When you exercise a lot, you tend to flush out acidic toxins from the body. Brisk walking ensures that your body removes waste more easily.

It isn't a bad idea to take a brisk walk daily, or if you are not a fan of brisk walking, you should consider adding a different type of cardio. Your body will thank you for this. You can easily get a friend, and before you can say, 'Jack Robinson', both of you are used to the routine. When you don't feel like brisk walking, your friend motivates you.

11. Raw unsalted almonds.

Almonds are the best things known to humanity, including almond milk. With the milk, you don't have to depend on high alkaline dairy milk that does more harm than good. When you eat a lot of almonds, the raw variety, your body is motivated to combat the acidity.

When you look at the nutrients that almonds have, you will notice that they possess magnesium and calcium. These are great in neutralizing the acid in the body. That's not all, as they help to balance out your level of blood sugar.

If you feel like snacking on something like cake or chips, toss the thoughts away, and go for unsalted almonds, and your body will thank you.

They help in reducing your hunger, and before you know it, the level of your pH is balanced.

12. Minimize the amount of sugar you consume.

Some foods that are high in sugar are very acidic. Examples are cakes, candy, and sodas. Everywhere we look at today, we see sugar, and sometimes, it is laced in the foods that we least expect.

Did you know that yogurt, ketchup and pasta sauce are all made with a lot of sugar? It is common to see several varieties of sugar in different forms. Sugar can be in fructose, corn syrup solids, high fructose corn syrup, dextrose, as well as sucrose.

It doesn't matter what form the sugar is in; they are all acidic. Now that you have realized that sugar is in almost anything you eat, you should consider eating a lot of alkaline foods, to balance out the effects of acidic foods.

If you want the pH of your blood to be balanced out, cutting down on sugar is the right way to go.

If you want to shed weight, and you are still consuming a lot of sugar-laced foods, then you have a long way to go.

13. Minimize your caffeine intake.

Almost everyone drinks coffee. You see people gulping it down every morning, and to them, their day isn't started without a swig of coffee.

Caffeine is seen in a lot of drinks that we access, especially in coffee.

What of the sodas that we drink? It could be your way of refreshing yourself in the afternoon when everywhere is hot. They may make you feel happy, but they aren't great for your health. Did you know that caffeine can increase the acidic level of your body, and before you know it, you will experience the side effects that come with an acidic bloodstream?

We know that you must take liquid. You can opt for tea or water.

14. Minimize the amount of stress you face.

Research has displayed that your emotions can determine the levels of your body's pH. When you are stressed, the neuron-endocrine system is affected. Once the system is affected, it could lead to cortisol increasing. Cortisol is a stress hormone that can increase your weight.

Many stressed people aren't actually aware that they are stressed. How can you tell when stress is occurring?

To help curtail negative effects, you should try to be mindful. Find out what is making you stressed. If you can, avoid it. If you can't, you have to devise a method of tackling it. Yoga can help.

When you nurture the mindful practice that works for you, you will be alert to the level of your emotions. Immediately after you notice that you are stressed, you should consider looking for a method to give you the needed inner peace. When you are at peace with yourself, the cortisol level reduces, and the acidic level clamps down.

15. Focus on consuming lots of high-alkaline foods.

Now that we have advised you to reduce the number of acidic foods that you consume, you should start consuming a lot of alkaline foods. This will leave your body in a higher alkaline state.

What you should consume are nuts, fruits, veggies, and legumes. Try out yams, sweet potatoes, eggplant, mustard greens and so on.

What is the link between the alkaline diet and cancer?

Over time, we have heard a lot of researchers say that acidic environments help stem the growth of cancer cells. This means that if you want to prevent the growth of cancer, you should consider eating alkaline foods and looking for methods to reduce the acidity of your blood.

Alkaline foods increase the pH levels in your body, which translates to your body becoming more alkaline in nature, reducing your risk of developing cancer. Many cancer survivors preach that eating foods that are high in alkaline can help.

Is it advisable for cancer patients to change their diets?

An alkaline diet can help prevent the risk of developing cancer, but it can't be said to cure cancer. Chemotherapy and other cancer treatments are known to be more effective in alkaline environments than acidic ones. Before you alter your diet, it is advisable to discuss with your physician or dietitian. This will allow you to know if it is good for the treatment that you are undergoing or not.

Before you change your diet, whether you have cancer or not, if you take pills of any kind, it is advisable to discuss it with your physician first.

When you discuss with your dietitian, he or she can look at what your nutrition goals are, and if changes have to be made at varying treatment steps.

The dietitian looks for ways to reduce the adverse effects that may come with any changes and see if you will face any food sensitivity.

With help from your dietitian, you can find out what diet works for you.

Chapter Five

Alkaline Recipes that you Should Try Out

While on your journey to embracing the alkaline diet, you should consider trying the following recipes. No one said you should eat only bland foods all in the name of being healthy. You can still treat your taste buds to great things in life, and enjoy healthy foods. This is what the alkaline diet offers. Gone are those days when you ate displeasing foods, all in the name of being healthy.

1. Green pea avocado spread

<u>What You Need</u>

    i.   Fresh green peas - Two cups

    ii.   One Avocado

    iii.   Green onion - Three tbsp. Minced.

    iv.   Lime juice - Two and a half tbsp

    v.   Himalayan salt - One-eighth tsp

    vi.   Black pepper- One-eighth tsp

    vii.   Chives – Chop and use for garnish.

Guidelines

Put every ingredient into the food processor and blend.

2. Traditional 'Beef' Stew Recipe [Vegan]

What You Need

   I. Olive oil - Two tbsp
   II. Garlic - Five cloves, minced.
   III. Onion - One, minced.
   IV. Tomato paste - Two tbsp
   V. White wine vinegar - One tbsp
   VI. Balsamic vinegar - One tbsp
   VII. Rice flour - Quarter cup
   VIII. Veggie broth - Four cups
   IX. Carrots - Two. Cut them into inch long pieces.
   X. Potatoes - Three and a half cups. Cut them into inch long chunks.
   XI. Celery - Three stalks. Cut them into inch long pieces.
   XII. Bay leaves - Three
   XIII. Black pepper - One Tsp
   XIV. Thyme - One tsp

XV. Parsley - Quarter cup

XVI. Beefless chunks - One and a half packs.

Guidelines

- Take out a big soup pot and put it on a stove on medium heat. Put in oil, allow it heat, stir in your onions. Allow it to cook for about five minutes.

- After that, stir in the tomato paste and garlic. Don't stop stirring until two minutes go by.

- Add your vinegar, and continue to whisk for a short time, before you stir in the flour. Don't stop whisking for about a minute.

- At this point, add in the carrots, broth, bay leaves, thyme, black pepper, and celery.

- Continue to stir, then reduce the heat to low, and leave it to cook for about forty minutes.

- While it cooks, don't forget to stir regularly to prevent the vegetables from getting stuck to the pan's bottom.

- Once the forty minutes are over, toss in the frozen beef, as well as the parsley. Allow it to cook for an extra two minutes, and you are ready to eat.

3. Lentil-Stuffed Potato Cakes

This is gluten-free and vegan.

<u>What You Need</u>

To make the cakes:

- I. Potatoes - ten
- II. Bay leaf - One
- III. Salt
- IV. Potato starch - One cup

To make the Stuffing:

- I. Olive oil - Two tbsp
- II. Onion- One, minced.
- III. Shiitake mushrooms - Four oz
- IV. Green lentils - Three-quarters cup. Cook them.
- V. Black pepper
- VI. Salt
- VII. Coconut oil

Guidelines

- Take out a big pot, and add bay leaf, potatoes, salt, and seven cups of water. Put on stove on medium heat, and allow it to boil until you notice that the potatoes have become soft.
- Use a fork to check if they are soft on the inside, and if they are, you know that they are ready. Once you are done, have the potatoes rinsed with cold water, as this allows the skins to peel off readily.
- Mash the potatoes until they are smooth, then stir in potato starch. Don't stop until they become a dough.
- If you notice that the dough is quite sticky when you attempt to shape it, stir in additional potato starch.

- It's now time to make the stuffing. Take out a sauté pan and place it on a stove on medium heat. Stir in onion, cook for about five minutes.
- Stir in mushrooms, then allow them to cook for an additional five minutes. At this point, toss in the salt and lentils. Allow them to cook for about two minutes.

- It is now time to make cakes. Take two tbsp of the dough and put it in your palm. Add the stuffing to the dough, fold it, and make it into a disk shape.
- Take out a skillet, and put it on a stove on medium heat. Put coconut oil in it, then add the potato cakes. Try to cook them until both sides have a golden-brown hue. Each side should take about four minutes.

4. Savoury Sweet Potato Breakfast Bowl

This meal is gluten-free and vegan.

<u>What You Need</u>

I. Olive oil - Half tbsp
II. Garlic - Two cloves, minced.
III. Spinach - Two cups
IV. Sweet potato puree - Eight oz
V. Pumpkin seeds - Three tbsp
VI. Sesame seeds - Two tsp

Guidelines

- Take out a medium skillet, and place it on a stove on medium heat. Put oil in it, toss in the garlic. Allow it to cook for close to a minute.
- Toss in the spinach, and allow it to cook until you notice that it is wilted. It should take an extra minute.
- Take out a bowl, and put the sweet potatoes in it. If you want to warm them, you should put them in a tiny sauté pot instead. Allow them to cook for about sixty seconds on a stove with medium heat.
- Add pumpkin seeds, spinach, pepper, salt and sesame seeds to the sweet potato.
- You can then serve. Enjoy.

5. Thai Green Vegetable Curry

What You Need

I. Vegetable stock - Two cups. Must be gluten free
II. Sweet potato - One
III. Thai Green Curry Paste - Two to three tsp
IV. Eggplant - One

V. Broccoli - One
VI. Zucchini - One
VII. Red bell pepper - One
VIII. Coconut milk - Two cups
IX. Kaffir lime leaves - Three
X. Fresh ginger – 1 inch knob
XI. Dash of lime
XII. Pepper
XIII. Salt
XIV. Coconut aminos - Two tbsp
XV. Jasmine rice.

Guidelines

- Take out a big pot, and place it on a stove on medium heat. Put the vegetable stock in, and allow it to boil. Toss in the kaffir lime leaves, chopped veggies, coconut milk, and grated ginger. Allow the mixture to simmer for about thirty minutes.
- Whisk it once in a while.
- After thirty minutes, add pepper and salt. Allow them to simmer for an extra ten minutes. Remove the pot from the stove.

- Toss the coconut aminos and lime juice into the pot. Don't stop whisking until they are fully combined.
- Don't forget to serve using whole grain jasmine rice.

6. High Protein Spinach and Rice Balls

<u>What You Need</u>

Part one:

I. Spinach leaves - Four and a half cups
II. Greek olives - One-third cup
III. Nutritional yeast - One tbsp
IV. Lemon juice - One tbsp
V. Garlic powder - One Tsp
VI. Salt - Three-quarter tsp

Part two:

I. Cooked rice - One-quarter cup
II. Almonds - Half cup
III. Chickpea flour - Half cup

To Serve Over:

Coconut yogurt

Guidelines

- Have the oven preheated to 360°F.
- Take every ingredient in part 1, and place it in the food processor. Allow it to blend well.
- Take out the mixture and put it in a big bowl. Put in the ingredients listed out in part 2, and mix well. Don't stop until you notice that it has the texture of dough.
- If you notice that the dough is too wet, put in extra chickpea flour. Avoid tasting it now, because when uncooked, it is sour. It is time to add the amount of pepper that you wish for.
- Use your hands to create twelve balls, then place them on a baking tray that has baking paper.
- It is now time to place it in the oven. It should take about twenty minutes. Sometimes, it may be twenty-five minutes. How you can tell if it is ready is if it doesn't have a bitter taste
- You can then serve them with coconut yogurt.

Lime and Coconut Panna Cotta

What You Need

I. Water - Half cup
II. Coconut milk - Half cup
III. Agar agar powder - Half tsp
IV. Lime extract - Half tsp
V. Agave nectar - Three tbsp
VI. Lime zest
VII. Berries or pineapples. Chopped.
VIII. Green food coloring. It is optional.

Guidelines

- Take out a saucepan, and put in the agar agar powder. Add a quarter cup of water to it, and allow it to sit for close to five minutes.
- Take out another saucepan, and put it on a stove on medium heat, then add the coconut milk. Allow it to warm.
- Take out the saucepan that has the agar agar, and place it on the stove on low flame.

- Immediately after it boils, put in the warm coconut milk. You can then add the remaining water, sugar, lime essence, coloring, and zest. Add every ingredient until they blend. You can then taste it to see if you need to add additional sweetener.
- Once three minutes go by, remove it from the stove, and place it in small bowls to sit. You can consume it at room temperature, but it tastes great when you leave it in a fridge to cool.
- You can then serve while cold, but top it off with berries and pineapple.

7. Onion and pepper masala

What You Need

I. Onion - One. Minced.
II. Bell pepper - One. Minced.
III. Garlic - Two cloves. Minced.
IV. Green chilis - Two. Minced.
V. Ginger - One inch. Minced.
VI. Cumin seeds - One tsp

VII. Tumeric powder - Half tsp

VIII. Cashew - One tbsp

IX. Asafoetida - Quarter tsp

X. Tomato ketchup - Three tbsp

XI. Garam masala powder - Half tsp

XII. Red chili powder - One Tsp

XIII. Vegetable oil - One and a half tbsp

XIV. Salt

Guidelines

- Take out a pan, and place it on a stove on medium heat. Add the oil, then allow it to cook for a while. Put in the cashews, turmeric powder, cumin seeds, and asafoetida. Allow it to sauté until you notice that they have changed to a light golden hue.

- Toss in the ginger, onion, green chilis and garlic, and allow them to sauté until the onion is translucent. This should take about eight minutes. While the onion sautés, toss in the salt. This allows it to cook quickly.

- At this point, stir in the red chili pepper, garam masala, and tomato ketchup. Allow them to mix well.

- Toss the bell pepper into the mixture, then as much water as you'd like. You can add more salt as well.

Allow it to cook for about five minutes, and the bell pepper will be done.
- You can serve it immediately.

8. Raw lemon meltaway balls

What You Need

- Almond flour - One and a half cups
- Coconut flour - One-third cup. Organic.
- Himalayan salt - Half tsp
- Maple syrup - Two tbsp. Organic
- Lemons - Three. Organic. Squeezed.
- Vanilla extract - Two tsp. Organic.
- Coconut oil - Quarter cup. Organic.

Guidelines

- Take out a food processor, and toss in every ingredient. Allow them to blend well.
- Use a spoon, and take some out. Put it on your palms and roll it. Do the same for the rest.

- You can either roll it in almond sugar or coconut flakes, or you can leave them like that.
- Allow them cool for about fifteen minutes in a refrigerator.
- Allow them to stay in the refrigerator, because if you remove them and do not serve, they can become soft.

Minced Tempeh Salad with Lemongrass, Sesame, and Cashews

What You Need

I. Lemongrass - Two stalks. Mince them after removing the hard outer layer.
II. Brown sugar - Two teaspoons
III. Sesame seeds - Two teaspoons
IV. Soy sauce - Two teaspoon
V. Lime juice - One teaspoon
VI. Chopped mint - One tablespoon
VII. Coriander - One tablespoon. Chopped.
VIII. Spring onions - Two

IX. Peanut oil to fry

X. Asian shallots - Five

XI. Cashews - One handful

XII. Garlic - Two cloves. Minced.

XIII. Fresh lime.

Tempeh

I. Tamarind - One and a half tsp

II. Tempeh - Three quarter cup

III. Brown sugar - One teaspoon

IV. Soy sauce - One teaspoon

V. Rice flour - One tablespoon

VI. Sriracha - One teaspoon.

Guidelines

- Take out a big skillet, and place it on a stove on medium heat. Put in about half an inch of oil. Take out two big plates, and place paper towels on them.

- Take out another small bowl, and add every salad ingredient, even the spring onions.
- Start to fry. Put the cashews in oil, and don't stop frying until two minutes go by, or until you see that they have a lightly golden hue.
- Use a slotted spoon to take them out to allow them to drain. Put them on paper towels to dry.
- Add the shallots, and allow them to fry for half a minute. You should remove them from the stove when you notice that they have browned, but they shouldn't be burnt.
- Have the garlic fried similarly for about thirty seconds. Take them out, and put on paper towels. Allow them to drain.

Tempeh

- Take out a bowl and add sugar, tamarind, sriracha, and soy sauce.
- Stir in the tempeh. Add rice flour, and don't stop stirring until they are coated well.
- In the oil, add the tempeh mixture, and don't stop stirring until it has fried well. This should take about

five minutes, and you will notice that it has a golden-brown hue.

- Use a slotted spoon to remove it from the pot, then put it on the paper towels to drain well.
- You can decide to add every component of the salad, or you can place them separately. Try and have them served with sriracha. Don't forget to add some chili slices, as well as a lime slice.

9. Spanakopita: Greek Spinach Pie

<u>What You Need</u>

I. Phyllo dough - Twelve sheets
II. Onion - One cup. Minced.
III. Garlic - Four cloves. Minced.
IV. Green onion - One cup. Minced.
V. Garlic - Four cloves. Minced.
VI. Sodium garbanzo beans - Fifteen ounces.
VII. Frozen cut spinach - Ten ounces
VIII. Kalamata olives - One-third cup
IX. Nutritional yeast - Two tablespoons

X. Tahini - One-third cup
XI. Lemon juice - Quarter cup
XII. Black pepper
XIII. Parsley - Two tablespoons
XIV. Oregano - Two tablespoons.

To do the Flaxseed Mixture

I. Lemon juice - Four tablespoons
II. Maple syrup - Two tablespoons
III. Flaxseed meal - Two tablespoons

Guidelines

- Have your oven preheated to 350 degrees. Take out a baking pan, and line it using cooking spray.
- Take out a skillet, and place it on a stove on medium heat. Put in the green onion, onion, two tbsp of water, as well as the garlic.
- Sauté it for five minutes, then add a tbsp of water to stop it from sticking. Cook until you notice the onions are translucent.
- Toss in the spinach, and allow it to cook for about five minutes. You can also remove it when the water has

been soaked up. As the spinach cooks, stir the lemon juice, flaxseed meal and the maple syrup in a bowl. Whisk them well until they are combined, then keep them somewhere to rest. Allow them to thicken. Toss in the rest of the ingredients, except the phyllo dough.

- Leave them to cook for an extra five minutes while on medium heat. Take them off the stove and place aside until they cool.
- Coat a baking dish with the flaxseed mixture.
- Place phyllo dough on it, as an extra sheet. Use the brush covered with flaxseed mixture to touch up on it. Do this for extra phyllo sheets.
- Spread the spinach mixture onto the pan. You can then spread the rest of the six sheets of phyllo dough. Don't forget to brush every one of them using flaxseed mixture.
- Place it in the preheated oven, and allow it to cook for about forty minutes. By then it should be golden brown.
- Have it cut, then serve.

10. Kale and golden beet salad

What You Need For The Salad

   I. Dino kale - One bunch
  II. Golden beets - Four
 III. Bell pepper - One
  IV. Carrots - Two
   V. Green Onion - Four

For Dressing

    I. Garlic - Three cloves
   II. Ginger - One inch. Peel it, and mince it.
  III. Canola oil - Two ounces
   IV. Apple cider vinegar - Two ounces
    V. Lemon juice - A dash
   VI. Tahini - Three tablespoons
  VII. Tamari - One tablespoon
 VIII. Dried oregano - Two teaspoons
   IX. Dried basil - One teaspoon

Guidelines

For Salad

- Take out a big bowl, and toss in the green onions and kale chiffonade.

- Have the carrots, beets and bell peppers grated. You can use your hand or try the food processor.
- Add the onion and kale to the grated veggies. Don't stop tossing until they mix.

For Dressing

- Take out a bowl and add every ingredient.
- Take out a hand-held emulsion blender, and use it to make the dressing.
- Add the dressing to the salad ingredients, then toss properly.
- Chill for at least an hour

11. Creamy lemon herb dressing

<u>What You Need</u>

I. Hemp hearts - Half cup
II. Lemon - One. Squeezed.
III. Chives – A few strands.

IV. Fresh dill – A few sprigs.

V. Fresh cilantro - A few sprigs.

VI. Garlic powder - One dash

VII. Himalayan salt

VIII. Onion powder - A dash

IX. Water - A third of a cup.

Guidelines

- Take out a blender, and blend every ingredient. Don't stop until it is smooth.
- Add water to the mixture a tbsp at a time. Continue until you get the consistency you want.
- Taste it to see if it has the flavour you desire. If not, add more of whatever ingredient you'd like.
- Chill before serving. It should make about five servings.
- Store the rest in a container that has an airtight lid in the refrigerator for up to a week.

Chapter Six

How to Start an Alkaline Diet plan

Have you decided to begin the alkaline diet plan, but you are wondering what to add?

If you've noticed signs of acid imbalance, it is important that you consume a large percentage of alkaline foods. Eighty percent would do the trick.

The other twenty percent can take the form of foods high in protein, as well as other acid-forming foods.

After you have noticed that the pH balance of your body is where you want it to be, you can reduce the amount of alkaline foods you eat. How do you know if the acidic content in your body has reduced? Take a urine test to test the pH level of your body. It can also be a saliva test. It is important to note that even if your pH level returns to normal, it can always increase again because the body produces acid, and the foods you eat can worsen the acidic content of the body.

This means that once your body has a balanced pH level, you still need to incorporate alkaline into your diet, but it can be reduced amount from 80% to around 65%. It is advisable to test to see the level of your pH regularly.

Below are some general tips to eating more alkaline:

- Opt for whole foods such as fruits, root crops, veggies, spices, seeds, nuts, beans, as well as whole grains. Avoid sugar, high carb foods and so on.
- Opt for alkalizing beverages like ginger root water, spring water, water with lime and green tea. This means that you will have to kiss other beverages goodbye or take them in reduced quantities.
- Take only small quantities of grains, fish, meat and pasta, as well as essential fats.
- Try to remove processed foods from your diet. Foods like white sugar, caffeinated drinks and white flour should go. They are acidic.
- Opt for the organic butter - the real butter. You can also try ghee butter, and if you want a hint of dairy in your life, use full-fat milk.
- Have your salads dressed using healthy fats like avocado oil, coconut oil, and cold-pressed virgin olive oil.

Sample day: Alkaline diet plan

To help you learn what makes up an alkaline diet, we have created a sample menu. When you consume these foods, you are sure to reach the needed 80% alkaline diet.

One thing that you should understand is that the diet is not geared toward limiting the number of calories you intake; nor does it want to completely remove foods. What it suggests is that you reduce the consumption of some foods like sugar to the bare minimum. It won't be a bad idea if you avoid those foods totally, but if you can't, reduce them as much as possible in your diet.

One thing that can't be seen in an alkaline diet is calorie counting. What is advised is that you consume a lot of alkalizing veggies and fruits. You should also restrict how you consume grains, meats, as well as processed foods, as they can increase the acidic level of your blood.

Breakfast:

Veggie scramble:

This will feed one person. You can increase the quantity to feed more.

What You Need

I. Eggs - Two
II. Green onions
III. Tomatoes
IV. Chopped Bok Choy
V. Bell pepper
VI. Any other leafy green you want.

Guidelines

- Crack the eggs and whisk them well. Ensure that your tomatoes, green onions, leafy greens, chopped bok choy and other ingredients have been washed and minced.
- Take out a pan, and place it on a stove over low heat. Add some oil, and allow your veggies to fry for few minutes before you add the eggs. Scramble them.

Serve With: **Ginger Tea**

Snack:

- Pear - One

- Toasted pumpkin seeds - One ounce.

For Lunch:

- You can opt for lentil soup, and add some streamed veggies. For the steamed veggies, try onions, carrots, kale, and broccoli.
- Try olive oil salad dressing on the steamed vegetables.

Another option for lunch is to opt for eating four ounces of tofu, tuna, chicken or hot salmon. Serve it with three cups of mixed fresh veggies like cucumbers, tomatoes, broccoli, carrots, and so on.

For the drink, you can opt for:

Lemon-dill vinaigrette.

For A Snack:

- Try a hard-boiled egg. Slice it and sprinkle minced parsley and sea salt on it.
- You can also consider snacking on celery, as well as carrot strips. If that doesn't want for you, try out red bell pepper strips.

- To some, almonds will do the trick as their snack.

For Dinner:

- Four ounces of turkey, chicken or fish, and add a baked sweet potato or yam to the meal. You can also add a mixed garden salad.
- Another option is to try out pasta that was made from quinoa, amaranth, or buckwheat. Avoid the one made from wheat. Top it using bitter greens like arugula or broccoli rabe. Don't forget to include almonds, zucchini, lemon zest and salt and pepper to taste.
- The side dish can be steamed zucchini with a hint of olive oil and garlic.
- You can decide to throw in a grated Pecorino Romano, though it is optional.

For seasonal fruits, you can opt for:

- When summer comes along, you should consider munching on grapes, cherries, nectarines or melons.
- When winter comes, you can try baked apples or roasted pears.

Chapter Seven

Is my favorite sauce alkalizing?

A lot of people ask if the sauce that they are crazy about has a high acidic or alkaline content.

One thing that should be noted is that every condiment that is added to a sauce can affect the alkaline or acidic level. This means that every sauce comes with a different alkaline or acidic content. Different hot pepper sauces, chili pastes, and even oyster sauces may have different pH levels.

When you start calculating their pH levels, there are some things that you have to remember concerning the metabolic effects that these condiments, sauces and so on come with.

Secrets in the sauce

If you want to know if a sauce is alkalizing or acidic, you should analyze every ingredient that is added to the sauce. Not every sauce is made with the same ingredients, meaning that you have to look at what products are added to them. Though sauces may come with similar names, what makes them up may be different based on the product.

It's important to know what kind of ingredients were used. Did you know that a sauce that has hints of the alkaline-forming apple cider vinegar doesn't come with a similar effect as one that was made from acid-forming white vinegar?

Did you know that the type of sweetener and the amount used can also alter its effects? Compare the effects of acid-forming white sugar to that of alkaline-forming whole cane sugar, and you may be surprised.

The way they are also made matters. Making them at home comes involves different methods than making them in a plant. A lot of homemade sauces tend to be better than those made in large quantities. For example, a pad thai sauce that is homemade is far better and alkalizing in nature that one that was bought at a grocery store.

Look at the entire picture

To see what the acidic or alkaline effect could be on your choice of food, you should analyze every ingredient, and see if it is alkaline forming or acidic forming in nature.

Try to see the quantity of each ingredient as well, as this allows you to know how much of an impact it makes.

Though the acidity or alkaline level of one food is important to know, you should find out what the total impact could be on your body when you eat all of the foods together.

Study the entire picture to have a glimpse of what you eat daily, and determine if it is alkaline forming or acid forming. Not every acid forming food should be avoided or restricted. Why, you may ask?

Though a food may be acid forming, it still may be a good addition to your meal plan. One example is walnuts. They may be acid forming, but they are great for the body.

As for the other acid forming foods such as sugar, they come with no value, and can be tossed to the trash can, or reduced to the barest minimum.

Look at the results daily:

Working on a balanced pH level is a daily affair. As much as we want you to eat a lot of alkaline foods, we don't want your bloodstream or body to be highly alkaline. What we want is a balanced pH of 6 to 8. The body already produces a lot of acids as it stands, just don't overburden it with more acid.

It is advisable to take pH tests regularly. What you should do immediately after you wake up in the morning is to test your first-morning urine pH. It allows you to analyze what the total metabolic acid load could be. It is important to know that what you consume can determine how your acid-base balance is affected. You can also see if your eating pattern should be altered.

If you aren't able to alkalize solely through foods because your taste in food doesn't change, you can also make use of alkalizing compounds.

Conclusion

Time and time again, we hear people lament that nothing they do can shed unnecessary weight.

They talk of how they have invested in fat slimming pills. According to these miraculous pills gotten off the shelf at a drug store or a supermarket, they can burn off the fat immediately.

Many of them ignore the fact that diet and exercise need to be incorporated.

They sell exaggerated facts and leave a lot of people trying to lose weight by pumping themselves with a lot of pills, yet nothing seems to be happening. Some people notice that, instead, they are rapidly adding weight.

What of those people that are exercising without watching their diet?

One time, I was at a gym with a friend, sweating it out on a treadmill, and my eyes wandered to a lady there, who was trying to lose weight.

She was exercising like the world would end that same minute if the pounds didn't disappear.

Later on in the day, after exercising, I decided to sit out at a café to watch the traffic going by and work on my book, and there she was.

She had a large burrito, the biggest smoothie they had, and chips on another plate. Before one could say, 'Jack Robinson,' she was done with everything and was already signaling to a waiter nearby. Another heap of chips came, she demolished them, and she was done.

My interest was no longer in my book, but on her eating habit. She was probably wondering why she had been exercising so long, yet nothing seemed to be working.

Losing weight is not a magical occurrence, where you merely have to utter some words, and the fats disappear. It is far from that.

You have to work for it. What you should do is eat healthily, try the alkaline diet. No one is saying that you should eat bland foods, far from it.

When I see some diets that force people to take tasteless meals, all in the name of shedding weight, I shake my head because I know it won't work.

The human body likes sweet things.

Eating bland foods for a while will prompt the body to crave those sweet things. Once the craving comes, you may be back to eating junk food before you know it.

What we advise is to cut down on those acidic foods drastically, and increase your consumption of alkaline foods.

You should also consider exercising to get a quicker result, and voilà, in no time, you will have the shape that you have always craved.

Thank You and have a nice life,

Laura Violet and Erika Sanders

Copyright © 2019

All right reserved. No portion of this book may be reproduced, stored in a retrieval system, or transmitted in any form or by any means – electronic, mechanical, recording or otherwise – except for brief quotation in printed reviews without the prior written permission of the publisher or the author.

Legal Notices

No part of this publication may be reproduced or transmitted in any form or by any means, mechanical or electronic, including photocopying or recording, or by any information storage and retrieval system, or transmitted by email without permission in writing from the publisher.

While all attempts have been made to verify the information provided in this publication, neither the author nor the publisher assumes any responsibility for errors, omissions, or contrary interpretations of the subject matter herein.

This publication is not intended for use as any source of advice such as legal, medical, or accounting. The publisher wants to stress that the information contained herein may be subject to varying international, federal, state, and/or local laws or regulations.

The purchaser or reader of this publication assumes responsibility for the use of these materials and information.

Adherence to all applicable laws and regulations, including international, federal, state and local governing professional licensing, business practices, advertising, and all other aspects of doing business in the US, Canada or any other jurisdiction is the sole responsibility of the purchaser or reader.

Printed in Poland
by Amazon Fulfillment
Poland Sp. z o.o., Wrocław